CHRONIC OBSTRUCTIVE PULMONARY DISEASE (COPD) MANAGEMENT DIET COOKBOOK

A Culinary Guide To Breathing Easier:

Nourishing Recipes For Lung Health-

Boost Your Wellness With Every Bite

DR. SHAYLA LEWIS

Table of Contents

DISCLAIMER

Write a brief complete Disclaimer for my diet cook book telling them that the author is not in any association with any company, business or individual and also this book is written by the authors knowledge and understanding

The information provided in this diet cookbook is based on the author's personal knowledge and understanding. The author is not affiliated with, endorsed by, or associated with any company, business, or individual. The recipes and dietary advice contained within this book are intended for informational purposes only. Readers should consult with a healthcare professional or a registered dietitian before making any significant changes to their diet or lifestyle. The author assumes no responsibility for any adverse effects that may result from the use or misuse of the information contained in this book.

CHAPTER ONE

Understanding COPD and its effects on daily life:

Chronic Obstructive Pulmonary Disease (COPD) is a progressive lung ailment that includes emphysema, chronic bronchitis, and refractory asthma. It is characterized by restricted airflow and persistent respiratory symptoms that have a considerable influence on everyday living. Millions of people worldwide suffer from COPD, which frequently causes dyspnea, chronic coughing, and an increased susceptibility to respiratory infections. These symptoms might interfere with daily activity, complicating even ordinary tasks.

Living with COPD demands adjusting to a new normal in which dyspnea and exhaustion may limit one's skills. This illness can have an impact on both physical and mental health. COPD patients frequently experience anxiety and despair as a result of the disease's restrictions and the uncertainty surrounding its progression.

Managing COPD effectively requires a multifaceted approach that includes both medical treatment and lifestyle changes. Understanding the condition and its effects on daily life is critical for patients, caregivers, and healthcare practitioners. Individuals can better manage their COPD by identifying the obstacles it presents and seeking appropriate assistance and resources.

The importance of nutrition in controlling COPD symptoms

Nutrition is essential for treating COPD symptoms and maintaining overall health. A well-balanced diet can improve lung function, increase immunity, and give energy for daily activities. However, COPD frequently creates special obstacles in maintaining appropriate nutrition. Reduced appetite, difficulties eating or swallowing, and higher energy expenditure from laborious breathing can all contribute to malnutrition in COPD patients.

Individuals with COPD should focus on nutrient-dense diets. Adequate protein intake is essential for maintaining muscle mass, which can help with respiratory function and physical strength. Furthermore, eating foods high in antioxidants and anti-inflammatory chemicals can help reduce inflammation in the lungs and relieve COPD symptoms.

Basics of a low-carb, antioxidant-rich, and anti-inflammatory diet

Several dietary treatments have been recommended to help control COPD, including low-carb, antioxidant-rich, and anti-inflammatory diets. A low-carb diet aims to limit carbs, particularly refined sugars and processed grains, which can cause inflammation and worsen COPD symptoms. Instead, it focuses on entire foods like veggies, lean protein, and healthy fats.

An antioxidant-rich diet contains foods strong in vitamins C and E, beta-carotene, and other antioxidants, all of which aid the body resist oxidative stress and inflammation. These nutrients are abundant in fruits, vegetables, nuts, seeds, and some oils.

Similarly, an anti-inflammatory diet focuses on foods that can reduce inflammation in the body, such as fatty fish high in omega-3 fatty acids, leafy greens, berries, and spices like turmeric and ginger. Individuals with COPD who incorporate these dietary ideas into their meals may find that their symptoms and overall quality of life improve.

There are a few prevalent issues and misconceptions about COPD management diets that should be addressed. A common myth is that all COPD patients should adhere to a rigorous, one-size-fits-all eating plan. In actuality, nutritional requirements might differ substantially between individuals depending on disease severity, comorbidities, medications, and personal preferences.

Another issue is the risk of weight gain linked with increased calorie and protein intake, especially among COPD patients who are overweight or obese. However, maintaining a healthy weight and enough muscle mass is critical for supporting respiratory function and general health in COPD patients.

Additionally, some individuals may be concerned that dietary limitations may make meal planning and preparation more difficult or costly. While some dietary approaches may include changes in shopping and cooking habits, there are numerous economical and accessible solutions available that can help with COPD treatment goals.

An overview of the cookbook's structure and how to use it successfully

The cookbook is intended to provide practical advice and delicious recipes tailored to the nutritional requirements of people with COPD. It is designed to address common issues and misconceptions while providing a diverse range of delectable and nutritious meal options. Each section of the cookbook focuses on a distinct nutritional approach, such as low-carb, antioxidant-rich, or anti-inflammatory, and the recipes are organized appropriately.

To utilize the cookbook effectively, readers should be familiar with the fundamentals of COPD management diets as stated in the introductory chapters. They can next look into recipes and meal ideas that are compatible with their preferences and nutritional goals. The cookbook offers advice on meal planning, buying, and preparation, as well as suggestions for adapting recipes to meet certain dietary restrictions or tastes.

Individuals with COPD who incorporate the cookbook's recipes and dietary ideas into their daily routine can improve their nutritional intake, better manage their symptoms, and improve their overall quality of life. Additionally, caregivers and healthcare practitioners can use the cookbook to assist COPD patients in their dietary journey.

An overview of Chronic Obstructive Pulmonary Disorder (COPD) and its types:

Chronic Obstructive Pulmonary illness (COPD) is a progressive lung illness that causes difficulty breathing. It is distinguished by airflow restriction that is not totally reversible. Chronic bronchitis and emphysema are the two most common kinds of COPD, and they frequently coexist. Chronic bronchitis is characterized by long-term inflammation of the airways, which results in a continuous cough and mucus production. Emphysema, on the other hand, harms the lungs' air sacs, diminishing their flexibility and causing shortness of breath.

Symptoms and development of COPD

COPD symptoms often start gradually and worsen with time. Common symptoms include shortness of breath, chronic coughing, wheezing, and chest tightness. As the disease advances, patients may experience frequent respiratory infections, exhaustion, weight loss, and swelling in their ankles, feet, or legs. In severe circumstances, COPD can cause respiratory failure and death.

Risk factors and frequent causes:
COPD is caused by a combination of causes, including smoking (the major cause), exposure to environmental pollutants (such as secondhand smoke, air pollution, and occupational dust and chemicals), genetic susceptibility, and childhood respiratory illnesses. Other risk factors include age, alpha- antitrypsin deficiency, and a history of asthma.

Importance of early diagnosis and treatment:
Early detection and treatment of COPD are critical for better outcomes and quality of life. Unfortunately, many patients with COPD do

not get diagnosed until the condition has progressed. Early detection enables prompt interventions to decrease disease progression, alleviate symptoms, and lessen the likelihood of consequences. Smoking cessation, pharmacological therapy (including bronchodilators and corticosteroids), lung rehabilitation, oxygen therapy, and influenza and pneumonia vaccinations are all possible management techniques.

Lifestyle Changes for COPD Patients

Lifestyle adjustments can help manage COPD and improve overall health. Quitting smoking is the single most critical step for smokers with COPD in slowing disease progression and reducing symptoms. Avoiding exposure to environmental toxins, such as secondhand smoke and air pollution, is also critical. A nutritious diet and frequent exercise can help COPD patients stay at a healthy weight, strengthen their respiratory muscles, and improve their general fitness. Furthermore, exercising excellent respiratory hygiene, such as appropriate handwashing and staying away from busy places during the cold and flu season, can lower the risk of respiratory infections. Finally, COPD patients should collaborate with their healthcare team to create a thorough management plan that is personalized to their specific requirements and objectives.

CHAPTER TWO
The Role of Nutrition in COPD Management

Diet has a significant impact on controlling Chronic Obstructive Pulmonary Disease (COPD) symptoms. Individuals with COPD frequently experience difficulty breathing and low energy levels, which can be influenced by their food choices. Certain meals might increase or lessen symptoms. For example, eating large meals or hard-to-digest foods may cause bloating and discomfort, making breathing more difficult. A well-balanced diet rich in nutrients, on the other hand, can help with lung health, increase energy, and improve general well-being.

Nutrients Required for Lung Health and Function: Several nutrients are especially necessary for sustaining lung health and function in people with COPD. This includes:

Omega-3 fatty acids: Found in fatty fish such as salmon, trout, and mackerel, as well as flaxseeds and walnuts, omega-3 fatty acids contain anti-inflammatory qualities that may aid in the reduction of inflammation in the airways, improving breathing in COPD patients.

Antioxidants include vitamins C and E, beta-carotene, and selenium, which protect lung tissue from damage produced by dangerous chemicals known as free radicals. Antioxidant-rich foods include fruits, vegetables, nuts, seeds, and whole grains.

Protein: Adequate protein consumption is critical for maintaining muscle strength, particularly in COPD patients who may develop muscle wasting owing to decreased physical activity. Lean meats, poultry, fish, eggs, dairy products, lentils, and tofu are excellent sources of protein.

According to some research, vitamin D insufficiency may be connected with worse COPD symptoms. Sunlight exposure and dietary sources including fatty fish, fortified dairy products, and egg yolks can help keep vitamin D levels stable.

Benefits of a well-balanced diet in COPD management: A well-balanced diet provides various benefits to people with COPD, including:

Improved lung function: Nutrient-dense diets promote respiratory muscle strength and function, resulting in greater breathing capacity.

Increased energy levels: Balanced meals provide the energy required to carry out daily activities and participate in pulmonary rehabilitation programs.

Optimal weight management: Maintaining a healthy weight puts less burden on the respiratory system, making breathing easier and enhancing overall quality of life.

Reduced inflammation: Anti-inflammatory foods can help reduce inflammation in the airways, potentially lowering COPD symptoms including wheezing and shortness of breath.

Importance of maintaining a healthy weight

Maintaining a healthy weight is critical for COPD patients since excess weight can aggravate respiratory symptoms and raise the risk of complications. Obesity increases strain on the lungs and diaphragm, making it difficult to breathe. In contrast, being underweight can damage respiratory muscles and reduce energy levels. A balanced diet and regular exercise can help you achieve and maintain a healthy weight, improve lung function, increase exercise tolerance, and minimize the frequency of COPD exacerbations.

Strategies for including healthful foods in your everyday meals:

Opt for nutrient-dense foods including fruits, vegetables, whole grains, lean meats, and healthy fats. These foods include vital vitamins, minerals, and antioxidants that promote lung health.

Plan your meals and snacks ahead of time to guarantee a healthy diet throughout the day. To meet nutritional demands, include a variety of foods from each dietary group.

Stay hydrated: Drink plenty of fluids, ideally water, to keep mucous membranes in the airways moist and aid with mucus clearing. Limit caffeinated and alcoholic beverages, as they might cause dehydration.

Cook and season your salads with heart-healthy oils like olive oil, avocado oil, and coconut oil. These oils include vital fatty acids without any harmful saturated or trans fats.

To limit sodium intake, flavor foods with herbs and spices rather than salt. Fresh herbs, such as basil, cilantro, and parsley, provide taste and nutrition to recipes while reducing the

Consider dietary supplements: In some situations, people with COPD can benefit from taking dietary supplements to address specific nutritional deficits. Before beginning any supplement plan, consult with your healthcare physician or a licensed nutritionist.

Individuals can improve their overall health outcomes by recognizing the importance of nutrition in COPD management and practicing healthy eating habits

CHAPTER THREE

Introduction to Low-Carb, Antioxidant-Rich, and Anti-Inflammatory Diets

Explanation of the Low-Carb Diet Principles:

A low-carb diet lowers carbohydrate intake, often by limiting processed sugars and starches and increasing protein, healthy fats, and non-starchy vegetables. A low-carb diet can help with COPD control for a variety of reasons:

Weight Management: Many people with COPD struggle to maintain a healthy weight, which is commonly due to a lack of appetite or increased energy expenditure caused by respiratory difficulties. A low-carb diet can aid with weight management by stabilizing blood sugar levels and increasing satiety, lowering the risk of obesity, which can exacerbate COPD symptoms.

Improved Lung Function: According to research, eating too many carbohydrates can cause inflammation and oxidative stress, both of which are bad for your lung health. Individuals who reduce their carbohydrate intake, particularly refined sugars and grains, may see an improvement in lung function and respiratory symptoms.

Stable Blood Sugar Levels: Blood sugar fluctuations can have an impact on energy levels and increase weariness, both of which are frequent in COPD patients. Individuals can maintain more stable blood sugar levels throughout the day by limiting carbohydrate intake and opting for complex carbs that are processed more slowly, resulting in prolonged energy and increased endurance.

The importance of antioxidants in combating oxidative stress:

Oxidative stress contributes significantly to the pathogenesis of COPD, causing inflammation, tissue damage, and reduced lung function. Antioxidants are chemicals that neutralize free radicals, which are unstable molecules that can cause cellular harm when in excess. In the context of COPD care, maintaining a sufficient antioxidant intake is critical for reducing oxidative stress and sustaining lung health.

Protecting Lung Tissue: The lungs are especially prone to oxidative damage because they are constantly exposed to ambient contaminants and respiratory irritants. Antioxidants including vitamin C, vitamin E, and beta-carotene protect lung tissue from oxidative stress, lowering inflammation and the likelihood of exacerbations in people with COPD.

Reducing Inflammation: Oxidative stress and inflammation are inextricably linked processes, one worsening the other. Antioxidants can reduce inflammation in the airways by neutralizing free radicals and blocking inflammatory pathways, which improves symptoms and slows disease progression in COPD patients.

Improving immunological Function: COPD patients are more vulnerable to respiratory infections due to compromised immunological function. Antioxidants have an important role in immune function by strengthening the body's defenses against pathogens and reducing the severity and duration of infections, lowering the risk of aggravation.

Understanding Inflammation's Effects on COPD

Inflammation is a defining feature of COPD, marked by continuous immune system activity and the production of pro-inflammatory chemicals into the airways. Chronic inflammation causes lung tissue damage, airway narrowing, and impaired lung function, all of which contribute to respiratory symptoms like coughing, wheezing, and shortness of breath. COPD inflammation is caused by a variety of reasons, including cigarette smoke exposure, air pollution, and respiratory infections.

Dietary Interventions Can Modulate Inflammation: While corticosteroids and bronchodilators are routinely used to treat inflammation in COPD, dietary interventions can also play an important role in modulating inflammatory pathways. Anti-inflammatory diets high in fruits, vegetables, whole grains, and healthy fats aid in the reduction of pro-inflammatory cytokines and promote a more balanced immune response.

The Effect of Inflammatory Foods: Certain dietary components can aggravate inflammation in COPD patients. These include processed foods heavy in refined carbohydrates and Trans fats, which cause inflammation and oxidative stress. Individuals can assist reduce inflammation and improve respiratory symptoms by consuming fewer inflammatory meals and focusing on nutrient-dense, whole foods.

Foods to include and avoid on an anti-inflammatory diet:

An anti-inflammatory diet focuses on foods that minimize inflammation and oxidative stress while avoiding those that increase these processes. The key components of an anti-inflammatory diet are:

Fruits and vegetables are high in antioxidants, vitamins, and phytonutrients, making them crucial for reducing inflammation and improving general health. Berries, leafy greens, cruciferous vegetables, and bright fruits like berries, oranges, and kiwi are especially useful to COPD sufferers because of their high antioxidant content.

Healthy Fats: Omega-3 fatty acids found in fatty fish, flaxseeds, chia seeds, and walnuts offer powerful anti-inflammatory qualities that help regulate the body's inflammatory response. Furthermore, the monounsaturated fats contained in olive oil, avocados, and nuts can help reduce inflammation and improve lung function in COPD patients.

Whole Grains: Unlike refined grains, which can cause inflammation, whole grains like oats, quinoa, and brown rice are high in fiber and antioxidants, which help to reduce inflammation and regulate blood sugar levels. Whole grains in meals can provide long-lasting energy and improve respiratory health.

Lean Protein: Lean protein sources include poultry, fish, lentils, and tofu, which contain critical amino acids for muscle repair and immunological function but lack the saturated fat and cholesterol found in red and processed meats, which can increase inflammation.

Individuals who adopt an anti-inflammatory diet should minimize or avoid:

Processed foods, such as sugary snacks, fast food, and packaged meals, are frequently high in refined sugars, unhealthy fats, and additives, all of which can contribute to inflammation and oxidative stress. Reduced consumption of these foods is critical for treating COPD symptoms and improving lung health.

Trans fats, which are found in fried foods, margarine, and many processed snacks, have been linked to inflammation and an increased risk of heart disease. Avoiding trans-fat-containing meals can assist COPD patients to reduce inflammation and enhance their overall health.

Tips For Meal Planning and Grocery Shopping

Meal planning and grocery shopping can be difficult, especially for people with chronic diseases like COPD. Here are some suggestions to make the process easier and more enjoyable:

Plan Ahead: Set aside time each week to plan your meals, taking into account your dietary preferences, nutritional needs, and COPD treatment goals. Each meal should contain a well-balanced mix of lean protein, healthy fats, complex carbs, and colorful fruits and vegetables.

Make a List: Before you go grocery shopping, make a list of the foods you'll need for your planned meals, as well as any pantry staples. Creating a list will help you avoid impulse purchases and ensure you have everything you need for healthy, balanced meals.

Shop the periphery: When exploring the grocery store, concentrate on the periphery, where fresh vegetables, lean proteins, and dairy goods are often found.

This is where you'll find most of the nutrient-dense, whole foods that make up an anti-inflammatory diet.

Read food labels and ingredient lists carefully, paying special attention to added sugars, trans fats, and artificial additives. Choose minimally processed foods with identifiable ingredients, and whenever possible, choose items labeled "low sodium" or "no added sugars".

Stock your cupboard with nutritious essentials like whole grains, canned beans, nuts and seeds, herbs and spices, and healthy cooking oils. Keeping these ingredients on hand makes it easy to prepare healthy meals and snacks at home.

Incorporating these ideas into your food and lifestyle will help you manage COPD symptoms, reduce inflammation, and improve overall lung health. Before making any significant changes to your diet, contact a healthcare practitioner or qualified dietitian, particularly if you have underlying health concerns or dietary limitations.

Getting Started With the Cookbook

The "Getting Started" chapter serves as the introduction to the Chronic Obstructive Pulmonary Disease (COPD) Management Diet Cookbook, giving readers a thorough overview of how it is constructed and arranged. The layout is intended to be easy to use and accessible to people with COPD and their caretakers.

The cookbook is often divided into sections that address various aspects of COPD control through food. These sections can include:

Understanding COPD-Friendly Foods: Explains the significance of specific nutrients, vitamins, and minerals in COPD management and emphasizes foods that are useful to COPD patients.

meals

Includes a variety of meals designed to fulfill the nutritional demands of people with COPD. Recipes are frequently organized by meal type (e.g., breakfast, lunch, supper, and snacks) and may include options for various dietary preferences and constraints.

Meal Plans: Provides sample meal plans that are balanced and tailored to promote respiratory health while also supporting dietary limitations and preferences.

Tips and Strategies: Offers practical tips on meal planning, grocery shopping, eating out, and dealing with typical COPD and nutrition issues.

Tips for Understanding Recipes and Meal Plans

Navigating recipes and meal plans can be difficult, especially for people with chronic conditions like COPD. To help readers make the most of the cookbook, here are some helpful tips:

Before you begin, read through each dish and meal plan carefully. Pay attention to serving sizes, ingredient lists, and cooking instructions to verify that meals match your nutritional needs and tastes.

Consider Nutritional Needs: When selecting meals and meal planning, keep the nutritional requirements for COPD treatment in mind. Look for foods high in protein, fiber, antioxidants, and healthy fats, which can aid with respiratory health and overall well-being.

Adapt to tastes and limitations: Feel free to change recipes and meal plans based on your particular tastes, dietary limitations, and ingredient availability. Substitute ingredients as needed and vary serving proportions to suit individual preferences.

Plan Ahead: Plan your weekly meals ahead of time to make grocery shopping and meal preparation easier. Use the cookbook's meal planning tools to build balanced and diverse dinners that promote respiratory health.

CHAPTER THREE

Essential Kitchen Tools and Ingredients

Providing your kitchen with the necessary tools and ingredients can make meal preparation easier and more fun. Some important kitchen appliances for COPD-friendly cooking are:

Sharp Knives: Using sharp knives to chop fruits, vegetables, and meats is easier and safer.

Nonstick Cookware: Nonstick pans use less oil and are easier to clean, making them excellent for cooking with little fat.

Food processors and blenders are excellent for pureeing soups, preparing smoothies, and chopping items fast.

Measuring Cups and Spoons: Measuring ingredients correctly is critical for following recipes and controlling portion proportions.

Slow Cooker or Instant Pot: These gadgets allow for easy meal preparation and can help tenderize tough portions of meat.

A COPD-friendly pantry should have the following crucial ingredients:

Choose lean protein sources such as poultry, fish, beans, lentils, tofu, and low-fat dairy products.

Whole Grains: Choose whole grains such as brown rice, quinoa, oats, and whole wheat pasta, which include fiber and important nutrients.

Fruits and Vegetables: Include a variety of colorful fruits and vegetables in your diet to acquire a wide spectrum of vitamins, minerals, and antioxidants.

Healthy Fats: Include sources of healthy fats like olive oil, avocados, nuts, and seeds to help your heart and lung health.

Herbs and Spices: Instead of using salt and high-sodium condiments, add flavor to your dishes with herbs, spices, and seasonings.

Meal Preparation Strategies for Busy Schedules

Meal preparation can be difficult, particularly for people with hectic schedules. Here are some meal preparation ideas that could save you time and energy:

Batch Cooking: Prepare large batches of staple foods such as grains, meats, and veggies ahead of time and split them out for convenient reheating over the week.

Freeze Extras: Place leftovers or excess portions of recipes in individual containers to make quick and easy meals on busy days.

Wash, chop, and prepare items ahead of time to save time cooking and assembling meals.

Use Convenience Foods Wisely: Incorporate nutritious convenience foods such as pre-washed salad greens, canned beans, and frozen veggies into your meals to save time while maintaining nutrition.

Plan for Leftovers: Use leftovers as a time-saving method by making extra portions to eat later in the week.

Setting realistic goals for dietary changes.

Setting realistic dietary objectives is critical for long-term success in controlling COPD with nutrition. Here are some tips for developing realistic goals:

Start tiny: Instead of attempting to completely alter your eating habits, start by making tiny, attainable modifications to your diet. Concentrate on one or two areas of improvement at a time.

Set clear and defined goals that are measurable and attainable within a realistic time span. For example, try adding one new COPD-friendly cuisine to your weekly meal plan or increasing your daily intake of fruits and vegetables by one serving.

Celebrate Progress: Recognize and celebrate your accomplishments along the path, no matter how minor. Recognize the good adjustments you've implemented and their impact on your health and well-being.

Seek Support: Ask family members, friends, or healthcare professionals to help you keep motivated and accountable as you work toward your nutritional objectives.

Be Flexible: Be willing to change your goals and techniques as needed based on your progress, preferences, and changing health requirements. Remember that dietary adjustments are not universally applicable, and what works for one person may not work for another.

Breakfast Recipes.

Breakfast is widely regarded as the most essential meal of the day and with good reason. A well-balanced breakfast is especially important for people living with chronic obstructive pulmonary disease (COPD). It sets the tone for the rest of the day by delivering the nutrition and energy required to power both physical and respiratory functions. In this chapter, we look at breakfast recipes that are specifically developed for COPD control.

Nutritious and Filling Breakfast Options

A nutritious breakfast is essential for people with COPD since it helps maintain energy levels and promotes respiratory health. Include foods high in key nutrients such as protein, fiber, vitamins, and minerals. To make well-balanced meals, choose healthy grains, lean proteins, fruits and vegetables.

Recipes:

Whole-grain pancakes with Greek Yogurt and Berries: Using whole-grain flour promotes digestive health and energy. Greek yogurt provides protein, while berries contain antioxidants and minerals.

Omelette with Spinach and Avocado: High in protein and healthy fats, this omelet is a satisfying meal. Spinach provides vitamins and minerals, including vitamin K and magnesium, that are useful to COPD patients.

Recipes for Sustained Energy

COPD care necessitates sustained energy levels throughout the day to support respiratory and physical activities. Breakfast meals should include slow-releasing carbohydrates, proteins, and healthy fats to keep energy levels stable.

Quinoa Breakfast Bowl with Nuts and Seeds: Quinoa is high in protein and complex carbs, providing long-lasting energy. Nuts and seeds include healthy fats and protein, keeping you satisfied and energized.

For a balanced breakfast, try whole grain toast with nut butter and sliced banana. Nut butter contains protein and lipids, but bananas are high in potassium, which helps control blood pressure and improve lung function.

CHAPTER FOUR

Understanding COPD and its effects on daily life

Chronic Obstructive Pulmonary Disease (COPD) is a progressive lung ailment that includes emphysema, chronic bronchitis, and refractory asthma. It is characterized by restricted airflow and persistent respiratory symptoms that have a considerable influence on everyday living. Millions of people worldwide suffer from COPD, which frequently causes dyspnea, chronic coughing, and an increased susceptibility to respiratory infections. These symptoms might interfere with daily activity, complicating even ordinary tasks.

Living with COPD demands adjusting to a new normal in which dyspnea and exhaustion may limit one's skills. This illness can have an impact on both physical and mental health. COPD patients frequently experience anxiety and despair as a result of the disease's restrictions and the uncertainty surrounding its progression.

Managing COPD effectively requires a multifaceted approach that includes both medical treatment and lifestyle changes. Understanding the condition and its effects on daily life is critical for patients, caregivers, and healthcare practitioners. Individuals can better manage their COPD by identifying the obstacles it presents and seeking appropriate assistance and resources.

The importance of nutrition in controlling COPD symptoms

Nutrition is essential for treating COPD symptoms and maintaining overall health. A well-balanced diet can improve lung function, increase immunity, and give energy for daily activities. However, COPD frequently creates special obstacles in maintaining appropriate nutrition. Reduced appetite, difficulties eating or swallowing, and higher energy expenditure from laborious breathing can all contribute to malnutrition in COPD patients.

Individuals with COPD should focus on nutrient-dense diets. Adequate protein intake is essential for maintaining muscle mass, which can help with respiratory function and physical strength. Furthermore, eating foods high in antioxidants and anti-inflammatory chemicals can help reduce inflammation in the lungs and relieve COPD symptoms.

Basics of a low-carb, antioxidant-rich, and anti-inflammatory diet

Several dietary treatments have been recommended to help control COPD, including low-carb, antioxidant-rich, and anti-inflammatory diets. A low-carb diet aims to limit carbs, particularly refined sugars and processed grains, which can cause inflammation and worsen COPD symptoms. Instead, it focuses on entire foods like veggies, lean protein, and healthy fats.

An antioxidant-rich diet contains foods strong in vitamins C and E, beta-carotene, and other antioxidants, all of which aid the body resist oxidative stress and inflammation. These nutrients are abundant in fruits, vegetables, nuts, seeds, and some oils.

Similarly, an anti-inflammatory diet focuses on foods that can reduce inflammation in the body, such as fatty fish high in omega-3 fatty acids, leafy greens, berries, and spices like turmeric and ginger. Individuals with COPD who incorporate these dietary ideas into their meals may find that their symptoms and overall quality of life improve.

There are a few prevalent issues and misconceptions about COPD management diets that should be addressed. A common myth is that all COPD patients should adhere to a rigorous, one-size-fits-all eating plan. In actuality, nutritional requirements might differ substantially between individuals depending on disease severity, comorbidities, medications, and personal preferences.

Another issue is the risk of weight gain linked with increased calorie and protein intake, especially among COPD patients who are overweight or obese. However, maintaining a healthy weight and enough muscle mass is critical for supporting respiratory function and general health in COPD patients.

Additionally, some individuals may be concerned that dietary limitations may make meal planning and preparation more difficult or costly. While some dietary approaches may include changes in shopping and cooking habits, there are numerous economical and accessible solutions available that can help with COPD treatment goals.

An overview of the cookbook's structure and how to use it successfully

The cookbook is intended to provide practical advice and delicious recipes tailored to the nutritional requirements of people with COPD. It is designed to address common issues and misconceptions while providing a diverse range of delectable and nutritious meal options. Each section of the cookbook focuses on a distinct nutritional approach, such as low-carb, antioxidant-rich, or anti-inflammatory, and the recipes are organized appropriately.

To utilize the cookbook effectively, readers should be familiar with the fundamentals of COPD management diets as stated in the introductory chapters.

They can next look into recipes and meal ideas that are compatible with their preferences and nutritional goals.

The cookbook offers advice on meal planning, buying, and preparation, as well as suggestions for adapting recipes to meet certain dietary restrictions or tastes.

Individuals with COPD who incorporate the cookbook's recipes and dietary ideas into their daily routine can improve their nutritional intake, better manage their symptoms, and improve their overall quality of life. Additionally, caregivers and healthcare practitioners can use the cookbook to assist COPD patients in their dietary journey.

COPD frequently experience difficulty breathing and low energy levels, which can be influenced by their food choices. Certain meals might increase or lessen symptoms. For example, eating large meals or hard-to-digest foods may cause bloating and discomfort, making breathing more difficult.

A well-balanced diet rich in nutrients, on the other hand, can help with lung health, increase energy, and improve general well-being.

Nutrients Required for Lung Health and Function: Several nutrients are especially necessary for sustaining lung health and function in people with COPD. This includes:

Omega-3 fatty acids: Found in fatty fish such as salmon, trout, and mackerel, as well as flaxseeds and walnuts, omega-3 fatty acids contain anti-inflammatory qualities that may aid in the reduction of inflammation in the airways, improving breathing in COPD patients.

Antioxidants include vitamins C and E, beta-carotene, and selenium, which protect lung tissue from damage produced by dangerous chemicals known as free radicals. Antioxidant-rich foods include fruits, vegetables, nuts, seeds, and whole grains.

Protein: Adequate protein consumption is critical for maintaining muscle strength, particularly in COPD patients who may develop muscle wasting owing to decreased physical activity. Lean meats, poultry, fish, eggs, dairy products, lentils, and tofu are excellent sources of protein.

According to some research, vitamin D insufficiency may be connected with worse COPD symptoms. Sunlight exposure and dietary sources including fatty fish, fortified dairy products, and egg yolks can help keep vitamin D levels stable.

Benefits of a well-balanced diet in COPD management: A well-balanced diet provides various benefits to people with COPD, including:

Improved lung function: Nutrient-dense diets promote respiratory muscle strength and function, resulting in greater breathing capacity.

Increased energy levels: Balanced meals provide the energy required to carry out daily activities and participate in pulmonary rehabilitation programs.

Optimal weight management: Maintaining a healthy weight puts less burden on the respiratory system, making breathing easier and enhancing overall quality of life.

Reduced inflammation: Anti-inflammatory foods can help reduce inflammation in the airways, potentially lowering COPD symptoms including wheezing and shortness of breath.

Importance of maintaining a healthy weight: Maintaining a healthy weight is critical for COPD patients since excess weight can aggravate respiratory symptoms and raise the risk of complications. Obesity increases strain on the lungs and diaphragm, making it difficult to breathe. In contrast, being underweight can damage respiratory muscles and reduce energy levels. A balanced diet and regular exercise can help you achieve and maintain a healthy weight, improve lung function, increase exercise tolerance, and minimize the frequency of COPD exacerbations.

Opt for nutrient-dense foods including fruits, vegetables, whole grains, lean meats, and healthy fats. These foods include vital vitamins, minerals, and antioxidants that promote lung health.

Plan your meals and snacks ahead of time to guarantee a healthy diet throughout the day. To meet nutritional demands, include a variety of foods from each dietary group.

Stay hydrated: Drink plenty of fluids, ideally water, to keep mucous membranes in the airways moist and aid with mucus clearing. Limit caffeinated and alcoholic beverages, as they might cause dehydration.

Cook and season your salads with heart-healthy oils like olive oil, avocado oil, and coconut oil. These oils include vital fatty acids without any harmful saturated or trans fats.

To limit sodium intake, flavor foods with herbs and spices rather than salt. Fresh herbs, such as basil, cilantro, and parsley, provide taste and nutrition to recipes while reducing the risk of fluid retention.

Consider dietary supplements: In some situations, people with COPD can benefit from taking dietary supplements to address specific nutritional deficits. Before beginning any supplement plan, consult with your healthcare physician or a licensed nutritionist.

Individuals can improve their overall health outcomes by recognizing the importance of nutrition in COPD management and practicing healthy eating habits.

CHAPTER FIVE

The importance of antioxidants in combating oxidative stress

Oxidative stress contributes significantly to the pathogenesis of COPD, causing inflammation, tissue damage, and reduced lung function. Antioxidants are chemicals that neutralize free radicals, which are unstable molecules that can cause cellular harm when in excess. In the context of COPD care, maintaining a sufficient antioxidant intake is critical for reducing oxidative stress and sustaining lung health.

Protecting Lung Tissue: The lungs are especially prone to oxidative damage because they are constantly exposed to ambient contaminants and respiratory irritants. Antioxidants including vitamin C, vitamin E, and beta-carotene protect lung tissue from oxidative stress, lowering inflammation and the likelihood of exacerbations in people with COPD.

Reducing Inflammation: Oxidative stress and inflammation are inextricably linked processes, one worsening the other. Antioxidants can reduce inflammation in the airways by neutralizing free radicals and blocking inflammatory pathways, which improves symptoms and slows disease progression in COPD patients.

Improving immunological Function: COPD patients are more vulnerable to respiratory infections due to compromised immunological function. Antioxidants have an important role in immune function by strengthening the body's defenses against pathogens and reducing the severity and duration of infections, lowering the risk of aggravation.

Understanding Inflammation's Effects on COPD:

Inflammation is a defining feature of COPD, marked by continuous immune system activity and the production of pro-inflammatory chemicals into the airways. Chronic inflammation causes lung tissue damage, airway narrowing, and impaired lung function, all of which contribute to respiratory symptoms like coughing, wheezing, and shortness of breath. COPD inflammation is caused by a variety of reasons, including cigarette smoke exposure, air pollution, and respiratory infections.

Dietary Interventions Can Modulate Inflammation: While corticosteroids and bronchodilators are routinely used to treat inflammation in COPD, dietary interventions can also play an important role in modulating inflammatory pathways. Anti-inflammatory diets high in fruits, vegetables, whole grains, and healthy fats aid in the reduction of pro-inflammatory cytokines and promote a more balanced immune response.

The Effect of Inflammatory Foods: Certain dietary components can aggravate inflammation in COPD patients.

These include processed foods heavy in refined carbohydrates and trans fats, which cause inflammation and oxidative stress. Individuals can assist reduce inflammation and improve respiratory symptoms by consuming fewer inflammatory meals and focusing on nutrient-dense, whole foods.

Foods to include and avoid on an anti-inflammatory diet:

An anti-inflammatory diet focuses on foods that minimize inflammation and oxidative stress while avoiding those that increase these processes. The key components of an anti-inflammatory diet are:

Fruits and vegetables are high in antioxidants, vitamins, and phytonutrients, making them crucial for reducing inflammation and improving general health. Berries, leafy greens, cruciferous vegetables, and bright fruits like berries, oranges, and kiwi are especially useful to COPD sufferers because of their high antioxidant content.

Healthy Fats: Omega-3 fatty acids found in fatty fish, flaxseeds, chia seeds, and walnuts offer powerful anti-inflammatory qualities that help regulate the body's inflammatory response. Furthermore, the monounsaturated fats contained in olive oil, avocados, and nuts can help reduce inflammation and improve lung function in COPD patients.

Whole Grains: Unlike refined grains, which can cause inflammation, whole grains like oats, quinoa, and brown rice are high in fiber and antioxidants, which help to reduce inflammation and regulate blood sugar levels. Whole grains in meals can provide long-lasting energy and improve respiratory health.

Lean Protein: Lean protein sources include poultry, fish, lentils, and tofu, which contain critical amino acids for muscle repair and immunological function but lack the saturated fat and cholesterol found in red and processed meats, which can increase inflammation.

Individuals who adopt an anti-inflammatory diet should minimize or avoid:

Processed foods, such as sugary snacks, fast food, and packaged meals, are frequently high in refined sugars, unhealthy fats, and additives, all of which can contribute to inflammation and oxidative stress. Reduced consumption of these foods is critical for treating COPD symptoms and improving lung health.

Trans fats, which are found in fried foods, margarine, and many processed snacks, have been linked to inflammation and an increased risk of heart disease. Avoiding trans-fat-containing meals can assist COPD patients to reduce inflammation and enhance their overall health.

Tips For Meal Planning and Grocery Shopping
Meal planning and grocery shopping can be difficult, especially for people with chronic diseases like COPD. Here are some suggestions to make the process easier and more enjoyable:

Plan Ahead: Set aside time each week to plan your meals, taking into account your dietary preferences, nutritional needs, and COPD treatment goals. Each meal should contain a well-balanced mix of lean protein, healthy fats, complex carbs, and colorful fruits and vegetables.

Make a List: Before you go grocery shopping, make a list of the foods you'll need for your planned meals, as well as any pantry staples. Creating a list will help you avoid impulse purchases and ensure you have everything you need for healthy, balanced meals.

Shop the periphery: When exploring the grocery store, concentrate on the periphery, where fresh vegetables, lean proteins, and dairy goods are often found. This is where you'll find most of the nutrient-dense, whole foods that make up an anti-inflammatory diet.

Read food labels and ingredient lists carefully, paying special attention to added sugars, trans fats, and artificial additives. Choose minimally processed foods with identifiable ingredients, and whenever possible, choose items labeled "low sodium" or "no added sugars".

Stock your cupboard with nutritious essentials like whole grains, canned beans, nuts and seeds, herbs and spices, and healthy cooking oils. Keeping these ingredients on hand makes it easy to prepare healthy meals and snacks at home.

Incorporating these ideas into your food and lifestyle will help you manage COPD symptoms, reduce inflammation, and improve overall lung health. Before making any significant changes to your diet, contact a healthcare practitioner or qualified dietitian, particularly if you have underlying health concerns or dietary limitations.

CHAPTER SIX
Getting Started With the Cookbook

The "Getting Started" chapter serves as the introduction to the Chronic Obstructive Pulmonary Disease (COPD) Management Diet Cookbook, giving readers a thorough overview of how it is constructed and arranged. The layout is intended to be easy to use and accessible to people with COPD and their caretakers.

The cookbook is often divided into sections that address various aspects of COPD control through food. These sections can include:

Understanding COPD-Friendly Foods: Explains the significance of specific nutrients, vitamins, and minerals in COPD management and emphasizes foods that are useful to COPD patients.

meals: Includes a variety of meals designed to fulfill the nutritional demands of people with

COPD. Recipes are frequently organized by meal type (e.g., breakfast, lunch, supper, and snacks) and may include options for various dietary preferences and constraints.

Meal Plans: Provides sample meal plans that are balanced and tailored to promote respiratory health while also supporting dietary limitations and preferences.

Tips and Strategies: Offers practical tips on meal planning, grocery shopping, eating out, and dealing with typical COPD and nutrition issues.

Tips for Understanding Recipes and Meal Plans

Navigating recipes and meal plans can be difficult, especially for people with chronic conditions like COPD. To help readers make the most of the cookbook, here are some helpful tips:

Before you begin, read through each dish and meal plan carefully. Pay attention to serving sizes, ingredient lists, and cooking instructions to verify that meals match your nutritional needs and tastes.

Consider Nutritional Needs: When selecting meals and meal planning, keep the nutritional requirements for COPD treatment in mind. Look for foods high in protein, fiber, antioxidants, and healthy fats, which can aid with respiratory health and overall well-being.

Adapt to tastes and limitations: Feel free to change recipes and meal plans based on your particular tastes, dietary limitations, and ingredient availability. Substitute ingredients as needed and vary serving proportions to suit individual preferences.

Plan Ahead: Plan your weekly meals ahead of time to make grocery shopping and meal preparation easier. Use the cookbook's meal planning tools to build balanced and diverse dinners that promote respiratory health.

Essential Kitchen Tools and Ingredients: Providing your kitchen with the necessary tools and ingredients can make meal preparation easier and more fun. Some important kitchen appliances for COPD-friendly cooking are:

Sharp Knives: Using sharp knives to chop fruits, vegetables, and meats is easier and safer.

Nonstick Cookware: Nonstick pans use less oil and are easier to clean, making them excellent for cooking with little fat.

Food processors and blenders are excellent for pureeing soups, preparing smoothies, and chopping items fast.

Measuring Cups and Spoons: Measuring ingredients correctly is critical for following recipes and controlling portion proportions.

Slow Cooker or Instant Pot: These gadgets allow for easy meal preparation and can help tenderize tough portions of meat.

A COPD-friendly pantry should have the following crucial ingredients:

Choose lean protein sources such as poultry, fish, beans, lentils, tofu, and low-fat dairy products.

Whole Grains: Choose whole grains such as brown rice, quinoa, oats, and whole wheat pasta, which include fiber and important nutrients.

Fruits and Vegetables: Include a variety of colorful fruits and vegetables in your diet to acquire a wide spectrum of vitamins, minerals, and antioxidants.

Healthy Fats: Include sources of healthy fats like olive oil, avocados, nuts, and seeds to help your heart and lung health.

Herbs and Spices: Instead of using salt and high-sodium condiments, add flavor to your dishes with herbs, spices, and seasonings.

Meal Preparation Strategies for Busy Schedules:

Meal preparation can be difficult, particularly for people with hectic schedules. Here are some meal preparation ideas that could save you time and energy:

Batch Cooking: Prepare large batches of staple foods such as grains, meats, and veggies ahead of time and split them out for convenient reheating over the week.

Freeze Extras: Place leftovers or excess portions of recipes in individual containers to make quick and easy meals on busy days.

Wash, chop, and prepare items ahead of time to save time cooking and assembling meals.

Use Convenience Foods Wisely: Incorporate nutritious convenience foods such as pre-washed salad greens, canned beans, and frozen veggies into your meals to save time while maintaining nutrition.

Plan for Leftovers: Use leftovers as a time-saving method by making extra portions to eat later in the week.

Setting realistic goals for dietary changes.

Setting realistic dietary objectives is critical for long-term success in controlling COPD with nutrition. Here are some tips for developing realistic goals:

Start tiny: Instead of attempting to completely alter your eating habits, start by making tiny, attainable modifications to your diet. Concentrate on one or two areas of improvement at a time.

Set clear and defined goals that are measurable and attainable within a realistic time span. For example, try adding one new COPD-friendly cuisine to your weekly meal plan or increasing your daily intake of fruits and vegetables by one serving.

Celebrate Progress: Recognize and celebrate your accomplishments along the path, no matter how minor. Recognize the good adjustments you've implemented and their impact on your health and well-being.

Seek Support: Ask family members, friends, or healthcare professionals to help you keep motivated and accountable as you work toward your nutritional objectives.

Be Flexible: Be willing to change your goals and techniques as needed based on your progress, preferences, and changing health requirements. Remember that dietary adjustments are not universally applicable, and what works for one person may not work for another.

Breakfast Recipes.

Breakfast is widely regarded as the most essential meal of the day and with good reason. A well-balanced breakfast is especially important for people living with chronic obstructive pulmonary disease (COPD). It sets the tone for the rest of the day by delivering the nutrition and energy required to power both physical and respiratory functions. In this chapter, we look at breakfast recipes that are specifically developed for COPD control.

Nutritious and Filling Breakfast Options

A nutritious breakfast is essential for people with COPD since it helps maintain energy levels and promotes respiratory health. Include foods high in key nutrients such as protein, fiber, vitamins, and minerals. To make well-balanced meals, choose healthy grains, lean proteins, fruits and vegetables.

Recipes:

Whole-grain pancakes with Greek Yogurt and Berries: Using whole-grain flour promotes digestive health and energy. Greek yogurt provides protein, while berries contain antioxidants and minerals.

Omelette with Spinach and Avocado: High in protein and healthy fats, this omelet is a satisfying meal. Spinach provides vitamins and minerals, including vitamin K and magnesium, that are useful to COPD patients.

Recipes for Sustained Energy

COPD care necessitates sustained energy levels throughout the day to support respiratory and physical activities. Breakfast meals should include slow-releasing carbohydrates, proteins, and healthy fats to keep energy levels stable.

Recipes:

Quinoa Breakfast Bowl with Nuts and Seeds: Quinoa is high in protein and complex carbs, providing long-lasting energy. Nuts and seeds include healthy fats and protein, keeping you satisfied and energized.

For a balanced breakfast, try whole grain toast with nut butter and sliced banana. Nut butter contains protein and lipids, but bananas are high in potassium, which helps control blood pressure and improve lung function.

Variations to accommodate various dietary preferences and restrictions

Individuals with COPD may have dietary preferences or constraints to consider while meal planning. Providing variety ensures inclusion and allows everyone to eat good breakfast foods.

Recipes:

Gluten-Free Breakfast Muffins: Made with gluten-free flour and oats, suitable for those with gluten sensitivities or celiac disease. They are loaded with fruits, nuts, and seeds for extra nutrition and flavor.

The Vegan Breakfast Burrito, made with tofu scramble, black beans, avocado, and salsa, is a great plant-based choice. It delivers protein, fiber, and important vitamins and minerals without sacrificing taste.

Tips for Quick and Easy Breakfasts

In the hustle and bustle of daily life, it is critical to have quick and easy breakfast options that do not sacrifice nutrition. These recipes can be made ahead of time or whipped up quickly, giving a stress-free start to the day.

Recipes:

For overnight oats, combine rolled oats, milk (or dairy-free substitute), and toppings like fruits, nuts, and seeds in a jar the night before. In the morning, grab and go for a quick breakfast.

Pre-pack smoothie components including frozen fruits, leafy greens, yogurt, and protein powder in individual freezer bags. In the morning, simply blend with the beverage to have a quick and nutritious breakfast on the go.

Importance of Beginning the Day with a Balanced Meal

Starting the day with a balanced meal not only supplies important nutrients but also sets a good tone for overall health and well-being. A well-balanced breakfast can assist COPD patients in maintaining their blood sugar levels, support lung function, and increase their energy levels throughout the day.

By emphasizing nutritious and full breakfast options adapted to COPD management, this chapter seeks to provide individuals with the knowledge and resources they need to start their day on a positive note, ensuring optimal respiratory health and overall well-being.

Lunch Recipes

Lunchtime may be a difficult meal to navigate, especially for people with Chronic Obstructive Pulmonary Disease (COPD). This chapter seeks to present a profusion of delicious and enjoyable lunch ideas that promote lung health while being convenient and easy to prepare. These recipes are not only healthful but also delectable, with a wide range of options to suit varied tastes and dietary needs.

Nutritious Recipes

One of the key goals of these lunch dishes is to ensure that they contain critical nutrients that promote lung health. This requires adding substances high in antioxidants, vitamins, and minerals with anti-inflammatory qualities. For example, meals with colorful vegetables like bell peppers, spinach, kale, and tomatoes are high in vitamins A, C, and K, as well as antioxidants that help fight oxidative stress and inflammation in the lungs.

Whole grains such as quinoa, brown rice, and whole wheat pasta are also high in fiber, which helps with digestion and promotes general gut health. Fiber-rich foods also aid with satiety, keeping people fuller for longer and minimizing overeating.

Portable options for on-the-go meals.

Individuals with COPD who live active lifestyles or have hectic schedules require portable meal choices. These recipes consider the requirement for ease and portability, providing foods that are easy to carry and eat while on the go. Wraps filled with lean proteins, such as grilled chicken or turkey, can be served with crisp veggies and hummus for extra flavor and nutrients.

Salads in portable containers with a variety of toppings, such as almonds, seeds, and grilled salmon or tofu, are also a wonderful option. These salads can be prepared ahead of time and refrigerated, providing quick and easy grab-and-go lunches without sacrificing flavor or nutritional content.

CHAPTER SEVEN

Incorporating lean protein and healthy fats

Protein is a vital macronutrient for people with COPD since it aids in muscle repair and maintenance. However, it is critical to choose lean protein sources to prevent consuming too much-saturated fat, which can lead to inflammation and worsen COPD symptoms. The recipes in this chapter use lean proteins including poultry, fish, tofu, and lentils, which provide plenty of protein without adding saturated fat.

In addition to lean proteins, these recipes include healthy fats to promote general health and satiety. Avocados, almonds, seeds, and olive oil are all sources of healthy fats, which contain important fatty acids that are good for your heart and reduce inflammation.

Strategies for Mindful Eating at Lunch

Mindful eating is an important element of controlling COPD since it raises awareness of hunger cues, portion sizes, and eating habits. Incorporating mindfulness activities during lunchtime might help COPD patients make smarter meal choices and prevent overeating, which can cause pain and worsen symptoms.

Here are some ideas for mindful eating during lunchtime:

Eating carefully and appreciating every bite: To avoid overeating, take the time to appreciate your meal's flavors and textures, as well as pay attention to feelings of fullness.

Portion control: Use smaller plates or containers to assist regulate portion sizes, and avoid providing enormous servings, which can lead to high-calorie intake.

Listen to your body: Pay attention to hunger and fullness signs, and stop eating when you're content rather than uncomfortable.

Minimizing distractions: Try to eat lunch in a peaceful, comfortable setting free of distractions like television or technological gadgets, so you can focus on your meal and completely enjoy the experience.

Individuals with COPD can improve their condition by implementing these measures into their mealtime routines. Furthermore, these lunch ideas offer a practical and delicious way to promote lung health while still eating satisfying and nutritious meals throughout the day.

Dinner is frequently the highlight of the day, with families gathering to share a meal and unwind after a busy day. Dinner can be an important component of the daily routine for people living with Chronic Obstructive Pulmonary Disease (COPD), giving not just sustenance but also an opportunity to enhance their diet and effectively manage symptoms. In this chapter, we'll look at delectable dinner options designed specifically for COPD management, with an emphasis on one-pot dinners, quick cleanup dishes, the use of veggies and whole grains, family-friendly ideas, and the significance of portion control and balance.

Flavorful Dinner Options For COPD Management

When creating dinner meals for people with COPD, it's critical to choose nutrient-dense products that can benefit lung health and general well-being. Lean proteins, such as poultry, fish, beans, and legumes, can offer vital amino acids without adding too much-saturated fat or sodium, which can worsen COPD symptoms. Furthermore, integrating herbs, spices, and low-sodium seasoning blends can improve flavor without relying on high-fat sauces or excessive salt.

Recipes such as grilled salmon with a citrus-herb marinade, turkey chili with beans and vegetables, and vegetable stir-fry with tofu are all delicious and high in vitamins, minerals, and antioxidants. These components not only help with respiratory function but also improve heart and immunological health, which are essential considerations for people with COPD.

One-Pot Meals and Simple Cleanup Recipes

For COPD patients, managing fatigue and conserving energy are critical components of daily life. One-pot dinners and dishes that need little preparation and cleaning can assist to speed up the cooking process and decrease mealtime stress. Casseroles, soups, and slow-cooker recipes are great choices since they allow for quick batch cooking and leftovers, reducing the need for regular meal preparation.

Recipes such as robust vegetable soup, chicken and vegetable quinoa casserole, and slow-cooker beef stew require little work and offer numerous servings, making them excellent for COPD patients and caretakers. These recipes highlight both respiratory health and practicality by using basic, nutritious ingredients and easy-to-follow cooking procedures.

CHAPTER EIGHT
Tips for Combining Vegetables and Whole Grains

Vegetables and whole grains are important components of a balanced diet for people with COPD because they include key nutrients, fiber, and antioxidants that promote respiratory health and general well-being. When creating dinner meals, it's critical to include a range of bright veggies and healthy grains to enhance nutrition and flavor.

Adding veggies to recipes like pasta primavera, quinoa salad with roasted vegetables, or vegetable and bean enchiladas improves texture, flavor, and nutritional value. Similarly, whole grains such as brown rice, quinoa, and whole wheat pasta include complex carbs that help maintain consistent energy levels and promote digestive health.

Family Dinner Ideas for Everyone to Enjoy

Managing COPD does not require losing flavor or enjoyment at meals. Dinner recipes that focus on healthful, tasty foods can appeal to the entire family while still satisfying the nutritional demands of COPD patients. Encouraging family participation in meal planning and preparation can promote a sense of community and support while also fostering healthy eating habits for everybody.

Recipes such as grilled chicken skewers with a vibrant vegetable medley, homemade veggie pizza with whole wheat crust, and shrimp and vegetable stir-fry are versatile and can be tailored to varied tastes and preferences. These dishes make dinner more pleasurable for everyone at the table by focusing on fresh, seasonal ingredients and adding a diversity of flavors and textures.

Maintaining portion control and balance is critical for COPD patients to maximize nutrition and effectively manage symptoms. Overeating can cause discomfort and worsen respiratory problems, whilst eating too few calories can cause weariness and weakness. Dinner dishes that focus on portion sizes and macronutrient balance can help people with COPD attain and maintain a healthy weight while also improving respiratory performance.

Incorporating lean proteins, whole grains, healthy fats, and lots of fruits and vegetables into each meal promotes a balanced intake of vital nutrients. Portion-controlled recipes such as grilled chicken breast with quinoa and steamed broccoli, lentil and vegetable curry with brown rice, or grilled vegetable salad with a side of whole grain bread give filling, nutritionally balanced meals that promote respiratory health.

Finally, supper recipes for people with COPD should focus on nutrient-dense products, easy preparation methods, and family-friendly options, while emphasizing portion control and balanced meals. These dishes, which include lean proteins, veggies, healthful grains, and savory seasonings, can help people control their COPD symptoms while also having wonderful, satisfying dinners with their families.

Snack and Dessert Recipes

Individuals with Chronic Obstructive Pulmonary Disease (COPD) frequently find it difficult to eat snacks and desserts. It is critical to achieve a balance between fulfilling appetites and following a diet that promotes lung health. In this chapter, we'll look at many tactics and recipes designed to address these needs.

Healthy Snack Options to Control Cravings: Snacking can either supplement or derail a well-balanced diet.

For COPD sufferers, choosing nutrient-dense snacks is critical to maintaining overall health and energy levels. Consider snacks high in protein, healthy fats, and fiber. Greek yogurt with berries, hummus with vegetable sticks, and a handful of mixed nuts are other examples. These foods provide consistent energy without generating blood sugar spikes, which can aggravate COPD symptoms.

Recipes for Satisfying Sweet Treats Without Sacrificing Nutrition: Satisfying a sweet taste while treating COPD necessitates culinary innovation. Fortunately, there are numerous delectable dessert options that can be both decadent and healthful. Try dishes that use natural sweeteners like honey or maple syrup instead of processed sugars. Consider making fruit-based sweets like baked apples with cinnamon or a refreshing fruit salad with a sprinkle of yogurt. These treats are a guilt-free method to satisfy cravings while also supplying necessary vitamins and antioxidants.

Portion Management Tips for Managing Snacking Habits: Portion management is essential for keeping a healthy weight and avoiding overeating, particularly when it comes to snacks and desserts. COPD sufferers should try to eat balanced quantities that give satiety while minimizing discomfort. To reduce mindless munching, consider preportioning snacks into individual servings. Furthermore, mindful eating strategies, such as eating slowly and paying attention to hunger cues, might aid in avoiding overindulgence.

Fruits and nuts are ideal complements to a COPD-friendly diet due to their high nutritional density and numerous health benefits. Fruits contain critical vitamins, minerals, and antioxidants, whilst nuts supply healthy fats and protein. Incorporate these items into snacks and desserts to increase nutrition and flavor.

Blend fruits into smoothies or add nuts to yogurt for a pleasant crunch. COPD patients can improve the nutritional content of their snacks and desserts by including these healthy items.

Mindful Eating Practices for Guilt-Free Snacks: Mindful eating entails being present and aware while eating, which can assist COPD patients in developing a healthier relationship with snacks and desserts.

Instead of eating on autopilot, relish each bite, focusing on flavor, texture, and scent. Mindful eating can also help you distinguish between actual hunger signs and emotional eating triggers. Individuals who approach snacks and desserts with mindfulness can enjoy them guilt-free and without jeopardizing their respiratory health.

To summarize, managing COPD does not imply giving up snacks and desserts entirely. Individuals can enjoy delectable snacks while improving their respiratory health by using the correct tactics and recipes. COPD patients can maintain a balanced diet without compromising taste or enjoyment by selecting nutrient-dense foods, practicing portion management, and adopting mindful eating practices.

CHAPTER NINE

Common Concerns and FAQs.

Addressing concerns about dietary limits and COPD: When managing COPD, people frequently worry about how their diet will affect their symptoms and general health. While there may be some dietary restrictions to consider, such as lowering sodium consumption to manage fluid retention or avoiding items that can aggravate symptoms like gas and bloating, it is critical to focus on a balanced and nutritious diet.

Encourage people to engage closely with a healthcare provider or a certified dietitian to assist them in negotiating any dietary limitations while still meeting their nutritional needs.

FAQs about specific chemicals and their effects on COPD symptoms: In this area, we address common concerns about how specific compounds may affect COPD symptoms. For example, many people are curious about the effect of dairy products on mucus production and respiratory function. While some COPD patients may find that dairy aggravates their symptoms, it is not a universal problem, and moderation is essential. Similarly, doubts may emerge over the efficacy of specific nutrients, such as ginger or turmeric, in reducing inflammation and improving respiratory health.

Tips for managing hunger changes and weight loss/gain: Individuals with COPD frequently experience appetite changes and weight fluctuations, which are generally caused by variables such as drug side effects, decreased physical activity, or increased energy expenditure from breathing. It can be really beneficial to provide practical ideas for dealing with these changes. For example, providing modest, regular meals packed with nutrient-dense foods can help people keep their energy levels stable without feeling overwhelmed. Furthermore, highlighting the necessity of staying hydrated and eating protein-rich foods will help muscle health and prevent accidental weight loss.

Strategies for dining out and social gatherings: Maintaining a social life and eating outside the home can be difficult for those with COPD, especially if they have dietary restrictions or respiratory problems. Providing solutions for handling these circumstances can help people participate fully in social events while managing their illness. This could involve reviewing restaurant menus ahead of time, picking places with sufficient ventilation, or ordering smaller servings to avoid feeling overly full or uncomfortable.

Setbacks are unavoidable when living with COPD. Here's how to deal with them and stay motivated. Whether it's a flare-up of symptoms, a slip in eating habits, or emotions of irritation and exhaustion, providing support and direction is critical for overcoming these obstacles. Encourage folks to set small, attainable objectives, use self-care techniques such as deep breathing or relaxation exercises, and seek support from loved ones or support groups to help them stay motivated and resilient on their path to better health. Furthermore, reminding people that setbacks are a normal part of the process and not a sign of failure might help them retain a positive attitude and sense of progress.

The importance of meal planning in COPD management

Meal planning is essential in the management of Chronic Obstructive

Pulmonary Disease (COPD) because it ensures that people with COPD get enough nourishment to support their overall health and well-being. COPD can drastically reduce an individual's appetite, energy levels, and ability to eat, resulting in weight loss, malnutrition, and muscle atrophy. A well-planned meal plan can help address these problems by ensuring that patients get the nutrition they need to stay strong and energetic.

One of the key advantages of meal planning in COPD management is that it allows people to predict their nutritional needs and make necessary adjustments. This is especially significant for COPD patients, who may have swings in appetite and energy levels throughout the day. Patients who plan their meals ahead of time can guarantee that they have access to nutritional foods that are simple to prepare, even if they do not feel like cooking.

Furthermore, meal planning might assist COPD patients in addressing specific dietary problems, such as avoiding items that can worsen symptoms or cause flare-ups. To prevent fluid retention and shortness of breath, people with COPD may need to limit their sodium consumption. Patients who plan their meals properly can choose lower-sodium options and have more control over their food intake.

CHAPTER TEN

Tips for Creating Balanced and Nutritional Meal Plans:

When establishing meal plans for people with COPD, it's critical to prioritize balance and nutrition. Here are some suggestions to consider:

Include a Variety of Foods: Incorporating a diverse range of foods ensures that COPD sufferers get the nutrients they need to stay healthy. Aim to include fruits, vegetables, whole grains, lean meats, and healthy fats in every meal.

Focus on Nutrient-Dense meals: Because COPD patients may have lower appetites, it is critical to emphasize nutrient-dense meals that provide a high concentration of key elements per serving. Examples include nuts, seeds, legumes, and leafy greens.

Consider Texture Modifications: Some COPD patients may have trouble chewing or swallowing, particularly during exacerbations. Consider changing the texture of foods to make them simpler to eat, such as pureeing fruits and vegetables or choosing softer, cooked dishes.

Portion Control: Pay attention to portion sizes to avoid overeating or undereating. Encourage COPD patients to eat smaller, more frequent meals throughout the day to stay energized without feeling too full.

Stay Hydrated: Proper hydration is vital for people with COPD since it thins mucus and makes breathing easier. Consume plenty of fluids throughout the day, including water, herbal teas, and broth-based soups.

Adding Variety and Flexibility to Meal Planning

Variety and flexibility are critical components of effective meal planning for COPD control. Here's how to include them in meal plans:

Experiment with Different Recipes: Encourage COPD patients to try new recipes and ingredients to make meals more interesting and enjoyable. This can help people avoid food boredom and keep them interested in eating.

Plan for Special Occasions: Make meal planning flexible enough to meet special occasions or social gatherings. While a nutritious diet is crucial, occasional indulgences can be part of a well-balanced eating plan.

Adapt to Changing Needs: COPD patients' nutritional requirements might alter over time, particularly during exacerbations or periods of illness. Be prepared to change meal plans as needed to ensure that patients continue to obtain proper nourishment.

Consider Cultural Preferences: When organizing meals, consider the COPD patients' cultural preferences and dietary habits. Incorporating familiar foods and flavors can improve mealtime enjoyment and satisfaction.

CHAPTER ELEVEN

Long-term Strategies to Maintain Dietary Changes:

Long-term dietary adjustments are crucial for optimal COPD management. Here are some techniques to promote long-term success:

Set Realistic objectives: Collaborate with COPD patients to create realistic and achievable dietary objectives that are tailored to their specific requirements and preferences. Break down major goals into smaller, more attainable tasks to help progress over time.

Provide Education and assistance: COPD patients should get continuing education and assistance to help them understand the importance of diet in controlling their illness. This may involve offering instructional materials, culinary workshops, or access to qualified dietitians.

Encourage self-monitoring: Instruct COPD patients to track their dietary intake and progress over time. This can help them recognize patterns, make necessary modifications, and stay inspired to continue making good choices.

Promote Lifestyle adjustments: Stress the importance of living a healthy lifestyle that goes beyond dietary adjustments. Encourage COPD patients to exercise regularly, reduce stress, and quit smoking to improve their overall health and well-being.

Recipes:

Egg and Vegetable Breakfast Scramble:

Scrambled eggs with bright vegetables like bell peppers, spinach, and tomatoes make for a protein-packed breakfast alternative.

Creamy Chicken And Vegetable Soup:

This soup combines succulent chicken, veggies, and a creamy broth to provide critical nutrients and hydration.

Salmon & Quinoa Salad:

Refreshing salad with flaked salmon, protein-rich quinoa, and fresh veggies, drizzled with a light vinaigrette.

Turkey and bean chili:

This protein-rich chili is made with lean ground turkey, kidney beans, tomatoes, and spices for a satisfying meal.

Spinach and Berries Smoothie:

Enjoy a nutritious smoothie with spinach, mixed berries, Greek yogurt, and almond milk for a refreshing and antioxidant-rich beverage.

Grilled chicken served with steamed broccoli and brown rice.

A well-balanced meal with grilled chicken breast, steamed broccoli florets, and fiber-rich brown rice can help manage COPD.

Tuna & White Bean Salad:
A protein-rich salad with canned tuna, white beans, cherry tomatoes, and cucumbers, tossed in a lemon-herb dressing.

Sweet potato and black bean quesadillas

Flavorful quesadillas with mashed sweet potatoes, black beans, bell peppers, and cheese. Served with salsa for extra zest.

Baked Cod and Herbed Quinoa Pilaf:

Flavorful quinoa pilaf with fresh herbs and vegetables complements tender baked cod fillets.

Oatmeal Raisin Energy Bites.

Energy bites made with rolled oats, almond butter, honey, raisins, and cinnamon are a convenient and energizing snack.

Day 1:

Egg and Vegetable Breakfast Scramble.

Snack: Greek Yogurt and Berries.

Lunch: Creamy chicken and vegetable soup.

Snack: Sliced apple and peanut butter.

Dinner: Grilled chicken with steamed broccoli and brown rice.

Follow a similar pattern throughout the month, ensuring a balance of lean proteins, whole grains, fruits, vegetables, and healthy fats. Encourage COPD patients to stay hydrated, consume antioxidant-rich foods, and eat smaller, more frequent meals to improve respiratory function and general health. Also, tell them to avoid excessive salt and processed meals, as these might exacerbate COPD symptoms.

Variations to accommodate various dietary preferences and restrictions

Individuals with COPD may have dietary preferences or constraints to consider while meal planning. Providing variety ensures inclusion and allows everyone to eat good breakfast foods.

Gluten-Free Breakfast Muffins: Made with gluten-free flour and oats, suitable for those with gluten sensitivities or celiac disease. They are loaded with fruits, nuts, and seeds for extra nutrition and flavor.

The Vegan Breakfast Burrito, made with tofu scramble, black beans, avocado, and salsa, is a great plant-based choice. It delivers protein, fiber, and important vitamins and minerals without sacrificing taste.

In the hustle and bustle of daily life, it is critical to have quick and easy breakfast options that do not sacrifice nutrition. These recipes can be made ahead of time or whipped up quickly, giving a stress-free start to the day.

Recipes:

For overnight oats, combine rolled oats, milk (or dairy-free substitute), and toppings like fruits, nuts, and seeds in a jar the night before. In the morning, grab and go for a quick breakfast.

Pre-pack smoothie components including frozen fruits, leafy greens, yogurt, and protein powder in individual freezer bags. In the morning, simply blend with the beverage to have a quick and nutritious breakfast on the go.

Starting the day with a balanced meal not only supplies important nutrients but also sets a good tone for overall health and well-being. A well-balanced breakfast can assist COPD patients in maintaining their blood sugar levels, support lung function, and increase their energy levels throughout the day.

By emphasizing nutritious and full breakfast options adapted to COPD management, this chapter seeks to provide individuals with the knowledge and resources they need to start their day on a positive note, ensuring optimal respiratory health and overall well-being.

Lunchtime may be a difficult meal to navigate, especially for people with Chronic Obstructive Pulmonary Disease (COPD).

This chapter seeks to present a profusion of delicious and enjoyable lunch ideas that promote lung health while being convenient and easy to prepare. These recipes are not only healthful but also delectable, with a wide range of options to suit varied tastes and dietary needs.

Nutritious Recipes

One of the key goals of these lunch dishes is to ensure that they contain critical nutrients that promote lung health.

This requires adding substances high in antioxidants, vitamins, and minerals with anti-inflammatory qualities. For example, meals with colorful vegetables like bell peppers, spinach, kale, and tomatoes are high in vitamins A, C, and K, as well as antioxidants that help fight oxidative stress and inflammation in the lungs.

Whole grains such as quinoa, brown rice, and whole wheat pasta are also high in fiber, which helps with digestion and promotes general gut health. Fiber-rich foods also aid with satiety, keeping people fuller for longer and minimizing overeating.

Portable options for on-the-go meals. Individuals with COPD who live active lifestyles or have hectic schedules require portable meal choices. These recipes consider the requirement for ease and portability, providing foods that are easy to carry and eat while on the go. Wraps filled with lean proteins, such as grilled chicken or turkey, can be served with crisp veggies and hummus for extra flavor and nutrients.

Salads in portable containers with a variety of toppings, such as almonds, seeds, and grilled salmon or tofu, are also a wonderful option. These salads can be prepared ahead of time and refrigerated, providing quick and easy grab-and-go lunches without sacrificing flavor or nutritional content.

Incorporating lean protein and healthy fats
Protein is a vital macronutrient for people with COPD since it aids in muscle repair and maintenance. However, it is critical to choose lean protein sources to prevent consuming too much-saturated fat, which can lead to inflammation and worsen COPD symptoms. The recipes in this chapter use lean proteins including poultry, fish, tofu, and lentils, which provide plenty of protein without adding saturated fat.

In addition to lean proteins, these recipes include healthy fats to promote general health and satiety. Avocados, almonds, seeds, and olive oil are all sources of healthy fats, which contain important fatty acids that are good for your heart and reduce inflammation.

Strategies for Mindful Eating at Lunch

Mindful eating is an important element of controlling COPD since it raises awareness of hunger cues, portion sizes, and eating habits. Incorporating mindfulness activities during lunchtime might help COPD patients make smarter meal choices and prevent overeating, which can cause pain and worsen symptoms.

Here are some ideas for mindful eating during lunchtime:

Eating carefully and appreciating every bite: To avoid overeating, take the time to appreciate your meal's flavors and textures, as well as pay attention to feelings of fullness.

2. Portion control: Use smaller plates or containers to assist regulate portion sizes,

131

and avoid providing enormous servings, which can lead to high-calorie intake.

Listen to your body: Pay attention to hunger and fullness signs, and stop eating when you're content rather than uncomfortable.

Minimizing distractions: Try to eat lunch in a peaceful, comfortable setting free of distractions like television or technological gadgets, so you can focus on your meal and completely enjoy the experience.

Individuals with COPD can improve their condition by implementing these measures into their mealtime routines. Furthermore, these lunch ideas offer a practical and delicious way to promote lung health while still eating satisfying and nutritious meals throughout the day.

Dinner is frequently the highlight of the day, with families gathering to share a meal and unwind after a busy day. Dinner can be an important component of the daily routine for people living with Chronic Obstructive Pulmonary Disease (COPD), giving not just sustenance but also an opportunity to enhance their diet and effectively manage symptoms. In this chapter, we'll look at delectable dinner options designed specifically for COPD management, with an emphasis on one-pot dinners, quick cleanup dishes, the use of veggies and whole grains, family-friendly ideas, and the significance of portion control and balance.

Flavorful Dinner Options For COPD Management

When creating dinner meals for people with COPD, it's critical to choose nutrient-dense products that can benefit lung health and general well-being. Lean proteins, such as poultry, fish, beans, and legumes, can offer vital amino acids without adding too much-saturated fat or sodium, which can worsen COPD symptoms. Furthermore, integrating herbs, spices, and low-sodium seasoning blends can improve flavor without relying on high-fat sauces or excessive salt.

Recipes such as grilled salmon with a citrus-herb marinade, turkey chili with beans and vegetables, and vegetable stir-fry with tofu are all delicious and high in vitamins, minerals, and antioxidants.

These components not only help with respiratory function but also improve heart and immunological health, which are essential considerations for people with COPD.

One-Pot Meals and Simple Cleanup Recipes

For COPD patients, managing fatigue and conserving energy are critical components of daily life. One-pot dinners and dishes that need little preparation and cleaning can assist to speed up the cooking process and decrease mealtime stress. Casseroles, soups, and slow-cooker recipes are great choices since they allow for quick batch cooking and leftovers, reducing the need for regular meal preparation.

Recipes such as robust vegetable soup, chicken and vegetable quinoa casserole, and slow-cooker beef stew require little work and offer numerous servings, making them excellent for COPD patients and caretakers.

These recipes highlight both respiratory health and practicality by using basic, nutritious ingredients and easy-to-follow cooking procedures.

Tips for Combining Vegetables and Whole Grains

Vegetables and whole grains are important components of a balanced diet for people with COPD because they include key nutrients, fiber, and antioxidants that promote respiratory health and general well-being. When creating dinner meals, it's critical to include a range of bright veggies and healthy grains to enhance nutrition and flavor.

Adding veggies to recipes like pasta primavera, quinoa salad with roasted vegetables, or vegetable and bean enchiladas improves texture, flavor, and nutritional value. Similarly, whole grains such as brown rice, quinoa, and whole wheat pasta include complex carbs that help maintain consistent energy levels and promote digestive health.

Family Dinner Ideas for Everyone to Enjoy

Managing COPD does not require losing flavor or enjoyment at meals. Dinner recipes that focus on healthful, tasty foods can appeal to the entire family while still satisfying the nutritional demands of COPD patients. Encouraging family participation in meal planning and preparation can promote a sense of community and support while also fostering healthy eating habits for everybody.

Recipes such as grilled chicken skewers with a vibrant vegetable medley, homemade veggie pizza with whole wheat crust, and shrimp and vegetable stir-fry are versatile and can be tailored to varied tastes and preferences. These dishes make dinner more pleasurable for everyone at the table by focusing on fresh, seasonal ingredients and adding a diversity of flavors and textures.

The Value of Portion Control and Balanced Meals

Maintaining portion control and balance is critical for COPD patients to maximize nutrition and effectively manage symptoms. Overeating can cause discomfort and worsen respiratory problems, whilst eating too few calories can cause weariness and weakness. Dinner dishes that focus on portion sizes and macronutrient balance can help people with COPD attain and maintain a healthy weight while also improving respiratory performance.

Incorporating lean proteins, whole grains, healthy fats, and lots of fruits and vegetables into each meal promotes a balanced intake of vital nutrients. Portion-controlled recipes such as grilled chicken breast with quinoa and steamed broccoli, lentil and vegetable curry with brown rice, or grilled vegetable salad with a side of whole grain bread give filling, nutritionally balanced meals that promote respiratory health.

Finally, supper recipes for people with COPD should focus on nutrient-dense products, easy preparation methods, and family-friendly options, while emphasizing portion control and balanced meals. These dishes, which include lean proteins, veggies, healthful grains, and savory seasonings, can help people control their COPD symptoms while also having wonderful, satisfying dinners with their families.

Snack and Dessert Recipes

Individuals with Chronic Obstructive Pulmonary Disease (COPD) frequently find it difficult to eat snacks and desserts. It is critical to achieve a balance between fulfilling appetites and following a diet that promotes lung health. In this chapter, we'll look at many tactics and recipes designed to address these needs.

Healthy Snack Options to Control Cravings: Snacking can either supplement or derail a well-balanced diet. For COPD sufferers, choosing nutrient-dense snacks is critical to maintaining overall health and energy levels. Consider snacks high in protein, healthy fats, and fiber.

Greek yogurt with berries, hummus with vegetable sticks, and a handful of mixed nuts are other examples. These foods provide consistent energy without generating blood sugar spikes, which can aggravate COPD symptoms.

Recipes for Satisfying Sweet Treats Without Sacrificing Nutrition: Satisfying a sweet taste while treating COPD necessitates culinary innovation. Fortunately, there are numerous delectable dessert options that can be both decadent and healthful. Try dishes that use natural sweeteners like honey or maple syrup instead of processed sugars. Consider making fruit-based sweets like baked apples with cinnamon or a refreshing fruit salad with a sprinkle of yogurt. These treats are a guilt-free method to satisfy cravings while also supplying necessary vitamins and antioxidants.

Portion Management Tips for Managing Snacking Habits: Portion management is essential for keeping a healthy weight and avoiding overeating, particularly when it comes to snacks and desserts. COPD sufferers should try to eat balanced quantities that give satiety while minimizing discomfort. To reduce mindless munching, consider preportioning snacks into individual servings. Furthermore, mindful eating strategies, such as eating slowly and paying attention to hunger cues, might aid in avoiding overindulgence.

Fruits and nuts are ideal complements to a COPD-friendly diet due to their high nutritional density and numerous health benefits. Fruits contain critical vitamins, minerals, and antioxidants, whilst nuts supply healthy fats and protein. Incorporate these items into snacks and desserts to increase nutrition and flavor.

Blend fruits into smoothies or add nuts to yogurt for a pleasant crunch. COPD patients can improve the nutritional content of their snacks and desserts by including these healthy items.

Mindful Eating Practices for Guilt-Free Snacks: Mindful eating entails being present and aware while eating, which can assist COPD patients in developing a healthier relationship with snacks and desserts.

Instead of eating on autopilot, relish each bite, focusing on flavor, texture, and scent. Mindful eating can also help you distinguish between actual hunger signs and emotional eating triggers. Individuals who approach snacks and desserts with mindfulness can enjoy them guilt-free and without jeopardizing their respiratory health.

To summarize, managing COPD does not imply giving up snacks and desserts entirely. Individuals can enjoy delectable snacks while improving their respiratory health by using the correct tactics and recipes. COPD patients can maintain a balanced diet without compromising taste or enjoyment by selecting nutrient-dense foods, practicing portion management, and adopting mindful eating practices.

THE END

www.ingramcontent.com/pod-product-compliance
Lightning Source LLC
Chambersburg PA
CBHW061046250726
48653CB00001B/283